Survival Skills

Basic Survival Skills Everyone Should Know

Table of Contents

INTRODUCTION

Congratulations on downloading *Survival Skills: Basic Survival Skills Everyone Should Know* and thank you for doing so. Inside this eBook are tips and tricks for surviving in the outdoors that you hopefully never need to use but should always know, just in case. The information inside this small reading holds the key to survival in some of the most dangerous situations you can find yourself getting stuck in.

Most rescues from the wilderness take on average 72 hours to locate and retrieve a missing person from their perceived danger. Although this is the case, surviving in the wilderness by providing your own shelter and food is not a dangerous situation with the proper knowledge and skills. The information in this book will provide everything you need to know in order to make sure the next time you are alone in the wilderness you are a self-sufficient individual thriving in a situation which others would consider dangerous.

It is important to note that individuals who push their limits in the outdoors also learn that limits push back. Although this book is full of survival tips to use while exploring, venturing out into the wilderness presents risks towards your safety and general well-being that the information in this book attempts to minimize, but do not eliminate. Hiking and other outdoor activities should always be with other individuals and never alone. It is important to always know your limits as a survivalist.

There are plenty of books on this subject on the market, thanks again for choosing this one! Every effort was made to ensure it is full of as much useful information as possible, please enjoy!

CHAPTER 1

PERSONAL PREPAREDNESS

To enter the wilderness, it is essential that you are first prepared with the proper knowledge and equipment of your surroundings. Entering the wilderness to hike a mountain in the northeast is significantly different than entering the wilderness to go rafting down the Colorado River. The most basic piece of equipment for the surviving the wilderness if the proper topographical maps.

Topographical maps are maps that indicate essential points of interest, landmarks, land formations and most importantly changes in elevation. Without knowing the topography of your given location, while trying to walk out of the wilderness you could end up attempting to walk up and over a mountain that is impossible to summit. In addition to providing the functionality of a regular map, topographical maps are drawn with contour lines that represent different levels of elevation. This is crucial for planning manageable goals for travel as well as locating water running downhill. Before entering the wilderness, it is crucial to practice and understand the functionality of your maps. The closer contour lines link together, the steeper the pitch of terrain. The proper maps are usually easy to locate. They are typically found at a parks office, outdoor supply store and even online.

In recent years GPS navigation has been increasingly popular. Global position systems are tools that use satellites to triangulate your location in order to tell where you are. GPS's have been decreasing in size in order to fit in the palm of your hand and can come preloaded with different trail maps and topographical information. Although these devices are increasing in popularity and functionality, it is important to note that they are not as reliable as traditional maps. They operate on battery power and have the potential to fail. When you enter the wilderness, it is important to not only know your surrounding and have the proper navigational tools but to also have backups in case you lose your map, or your GPS fails.

All maps are only functional with a compass. A compass works by using the earth's magnetic poles to pull its needle due north. Without this tool, your map is unusable since you would not be able to follow the maps cardinal directions. If your compass is destroyed or lost, there are still several methods for still finding your direction.

The first would be to make your own compass. To do this you will need a bowl of water, a magnet, cork (or anything that floats well above water), and a needle or screw. These items could be hard to locate in your pack of supplies, but if you prepare properly these are light weight and easy to store. Firstly, you will have to magnetize your needle by rubbing it against your magnet until it receives a proper magnetic charge. Next, you will push the needle through the piece of cork and place it in the middle of your bowl of water. If the needle is magnetized properly, one end will point north and the other will point south once it settles in the bowl of water.

The earth's magnetic field will pull the largest end of the needle north and the shorter end south. If the needle is not magnetized properly, it will float aimlessly without direction and you will be able to settle it in any direction. This is an effective method for establishing due north if you have the materials at your disposal and a flat surface to rest your bowl of water on.

If you do not have a piece of cork you can also make a similar compass with a pencil, magnet, needle, fishing line, and a cup. This is a similar process but instead of putting your magnetized needle through a piece of cork, tie it to your pencil, place the pencil over the rim of your cup to let the needle hang freely so the magnetic sphere can pull the needle north.

If you cannot locate these items, you can also use the sun several ways to identify cardinal directions. Other than knowing that the sun rises in the east and sets in the west, you can tell the direction during any time of day with the proper understanding of the suns movement in the sky. The sun moves in different paths in the sky depending on the time of year. In the northern hemispheres, the sun takes a shorter path in the sky and reaches a lower zenith (the point the sun is highest in the sky) in the winter months than the summer months. During summer in the northern hemisphere, the sun rises east due north; in the winter it rises east due south.

To locate direction at any time of year and day, you can use an analog watch. This method is only an approximate measurement and depends on the time of your watch being accurate. To do this in the northern hemisphere, point the hour hand of your watch directly at the sun and regardless of the time of day, halfway between the hour hand and the twelve o'clock mark points south. When attempting this in the southern hemisphere this would indicate the opposite: north. This method should only be used as a method of last resort since this can be relatively arbitrary with a smaller watch face.

If you do not have an analog watch, you can use any stick about a meter high. First, place the stick in a flat sunny area, so that you are able to identify its shadow. Once it is standing at a 90-degree angle mark the tip of its shadow with a stone. Wait for the sun to move in the sky for about ten to twenty minutes and then place another stone at the new location at the tips of the sun rods shadow. No matter where you are in the world, the first shadow will be in the direction of due west and the second shadow will be in the direction of due east. If you place your right foot on the second mark and your left foot on the first mark, so your back is to the sun rod, you are now facing due north and due south is directly behind you. This method can be used anywhere and requires no additional equipment. Although this is very convenient, this should not be rushed. The longer you wait between marking the second location, the more accurate your results will be.

Surviving the wilderness requires much more equipment other than the proper navigational tools. One of the most important pieces of equipment you can purchase for survival away from civilization is the right backpack.

Choosing the right pack is an intimidating experience that requires your full attention. If you plan to spend any longer in the wilderness than a day trip, you are going to want to purchase a frame pack. Frame packs are larger sized backpacks that have metal structures in them to give the bag shape and rest more comfortably on your shoulders. Frames are either internal or external. Internal frames are larger and provided more space on the inside of the pack. Although external frames do not provide as much internal storage, they typically provide more opportunities for lash points along the bag for opportunities to tie equipment on.

If you plan to spend 1-3 nights in the wilderness a "weekender" pack should be big enough for you. A weekender is a pack that typically has 30 to 50 liters of free space to pack your essentials. A multiday backpack is for the survivalist who plans to spend 3-5 nights in the wilderness and needs 50-70 liters of room to pack their survival gear. If you plan to spend an extended trip away from civilization longer than a week you may require something even larger.

Fittings for the proper backpack are usually conducted in specialty outdoor retailers. Most professionals will use a ratio of torso length and waist size to calculate the perfect fitting backpack for your specific build. There are also packs specific for women and children that reflect different shaped bodies.

When purchasing your backpack, it is important to consider what you realistically will pack in it. It is always essential to pack items for when disaster strikes like extra food and a medical kit, but you do not want to be carrying more than you have to. There are endless kinds of different features on the latest backpacks that you have to consider for different kinds of storage. Don't be shy with your purchase and be sure to consult your outdoor retailer on the bag that has the most applicable features and fit.

In terms of outfitting your clothing for the wilderness, there are several big mistakes, the biggest being cotton. Of all the options available for clothing material, cotton is the worst possible choice for entering the wilderness. The clothes we wear do not actually warm our bodies, they only insulate the heat that our bodies already make. Cotton is filled with air pockets that are vulnerable to absorbing and holding water.

When cotton gets wet, it stays wet since it cannot escape from the air pockets of its thick fibers. Unfortunately, this destroys cotton's ability to insulate our bodies. If it is colder outside than the temperature of your body, you will feel cold if you perspired in a cotton T-shirt. This can be dangerous since it does not have to be below freezing for a human to experience hypothermia. Wearing clothing like cotton that is porous and retains sweat can end up being life-threatening over time.

To properly outfit for outdoor survival you will need clothing made from quick drying materials that also lets your body heat and cool naturally. To eliminate the danger of wet clothing layers will provide a safety net. In the event that you are getting wet from overheating and perspiration, it is always effective to take off and put layers on accordingly. Overheating and sweating into a shirt all day can prove to be fatal if you only have that shirt to wear when it gets cold at night. Although brands like Patagonia and The North Face are expensive, they offer products that work well in layered systems and do not retain water.

One of the most overlooked pieces of essential equipment is the proper socks. When surviving in the wilderness you will be required to constantly be on your feet which will be vulnerable to blistering. A survivalist experiencing blistered feet will be in extreme pain and potentially lose their ability to walk. Be sure to wear thick wool socks or other products that specifically prevent blisters.

When packing extra clothes do not forget to leave space for an appropriate amount of provisions for the wilderness if you are not confident enough to hunt and trap your own food. The food you choose to bring should be both based on weight and amount of energy it will give you. For example granola, protein bars, and rice are light-weight foods that provide a quality amount of energy. Canned foods like soup might seem convenient, but they are heavy and do not provide as much nutritional value. No matter how you get your food in the wilderness, you want to be eating as much as you can at a realistic rate before you exit or are rescued. Food storage plans that involve fasting over a period of time and eating during another, have been proven not to work.

When surviving in the wilderness it is essential that you maintain a state of physical and mental alertness that is not maintainable while fasting. As a rule of thumb, always pack an extra day worth of food.

The items in your backpack should also have an adequate amount of comfort items that reflect your level of survival abilities. If you are not confident in your fire-starting abilities, be sure to pack a lighter or flint; if you are not skilled in making shelter, you should obviously pack a tent. Preparation for the wilderness is key to survival. Packing less and going light-weight is always an attractive option but be sure to always pack important items like your med kit and flashlight.

CHAPTER 2

BUILDING A CAMPSITE

One of the most important skills for survival is constructing shelter. Your shelter should be functional in terms of the climate around you and your expectations for how that climate might change. When deciding what type of shelter to make, it is important to consider how much time and labor it will require. This is frequently overlooked. Although it is often important to make a shelter to certain specifications, sometimes factors like daylight and approaching weather will force you to make compromises with your shelter construction. Your semi-permanent shelter should also always be constructed with the impression that your environments conditions will only get worse.

Choose a location: First things first, when it comes to creating a camp you can rely on, you are going to want to choose the best location possible. Above all else, this means choosing a safe location that is away from locations that might be frequented by predators as well as away from any natural impediments to your safety. You should also aim for someplace that is visible from above incase an airplane happens by. If this is the case, then you will need to be especially aware of thunderstorms as you could end up being the highest point in the area. You will also do will to choose a spot that has the best sightlines around.

Basic shelter: If you find yourself out in the wild without a tent, the first thing you are going to need to consider is a way to raise yourself up off the ground for the night. Not only will this keep you warmer, the ground sucks a surprising amount of heat, it will also protect you from all manner of crawling bugs plus all the things that eat those bugs as well. If you have food, you are also going to want to be sure that you keep it far away from the rest of your camp and as thoroughly out of the reach of animals as possible. Remember, you never know how long you are going to need to make your food last, don't share it any more than you have to. Remember, many animals are naturally wary of unfamiliar smells which means that if you urinate around the perimeter of your camp you will have fewer unwanted visitors. Finally, when it comes to taking care of bodily functions it is important to choose a spot to defecate that is at least 50 feet downwind from your camp and to always bury your leavings to avoid attracting animals.

Build a lean-to: When you are in a hurry to beat the sun down and are rushed by other elements of nature, the lean-to is the most practical construction. A lean-to is a three-sided enclosure that takes minimal labor and time to construct. It is constructed by finding two strong trees that are small in diameter and spaced out by 7-10 feet. Then fasten a tree branch horizontally between the two about three feet off the ground, this will be your base. To fasten this base together you will want to use a series of weeds, vines and emergency rope to make this as strong as possible since it will be holding a large sum of weight. Once the base is secure, start piling sticks on top of your base creating the triangular roof of your lean-to. You can further insulate your lean-to with leaves on the tops and sides of it. This is not the strongest type of shelter you can construct in the wilderness, but it is one of the easiest ones to make and offers light protection from the wind and rain.

If you are in a cold, wet environment, then you may want to create a fire pit underneath your lean-to, especially if you don't have a lot of other options when it comes to warmth. It is important to avoid this in most climates, however, as it is likely that your lean-to will become a fire hazard quite quickly otherwise. If you are planning on putting your fire pit in your lean-to it is important to build it with this in mind from the start. Position the firepit near the opening of the lean-to in order to ensure it has the ventilation it needs as well.

Take it up a notch: A more reliable, but labor-intensive shelter would be a grass thatched wickiup. A wickiup is an American Indian styled shelter that has a circular frame constructed from strong branches. If you are in a desert setting or have grass/straw at your disposal, a wickiup is easy to insulate.

Construction for a wickiup starts with burying three posts at least 12 inches deep in the earth and arranging them to stand together freely so they look like a pyramid. Once you have secured your first, and strongest posts draw a circle that connects all three posts. Take your time doing this and make sure it is an adequate size because it will be the blueprint for your soon to be shelter. Continue adding branches of similar height around the circumference of the circle but be sure to leave a section open for an adequate sized door. The strongest wickiups are the large ones that have strong posts securely grounded in the earth. To insulate this shelter (or any shelter) you will need to sandwich a layer of leaves, grass, hay or straw between your base layer of supports and a smaller lighter layer of branches above it. When you have settled in your shelter and would like to improve its structure, weave your top layer of branches in and out of each other in a way that they hold shape and the insulation cannot escape. This shelter is highly reliable against wind and rain when the time has been taken to properly support and insulate it.

All shelters can be improved once they have been constructed. The first luxury usually added to a shelter is a fireplace for warmth. It is important to remember that a fireplace is always an extension of a shelter and should not be inserted in an already established place for living. This is because most shelters constructed in the wilderness are built out of flammable materials. If your shelter is insulated with hay you should only include a fireplace if you construct an adequate addition to your already existing living space. Your fire will need room to breathe and ventilate in a space that does not compete for room with your body.

If you are surviving in a mountainous setting the most reliable shelters are rock shelters or caves. Obviously, this natural shelter does not need construction and has many strengths. If you choose a cave shelter for your survival setting, it is important to still keep in mind it will need insulation. Even in a large open area, we are able to trap our body heat a similar way the clothes on our bodies do. A cave might seem like an easy solution, but without proper insulation, the inside of a cave typically is colder than the area around it due to a lack of sunlight.

It is a common mistake to overlook this and not plan accordingly with either proper insulation or a ventilated place for a fire.

A key part of your shelter would be an adequate bed or sleeping mat. This is an easier construction than you would think that can be made with materials that are abundant all year. Dry grass is the most obvious material that is usually found at the base of cliffs that retain sun exposure. Small twigs and thin branches, much like a bird's nest, can be gathered and bundled neatly to make adequate bedding in the wild. Tying together a range of different gathered materials that you would use for insulation work well as a mattress. This is an important construction, not just for comfort, but to protect your body from the cold ground. Without the proper mattress, you would run the risk of sickness from the cold in the night.

Making fire: It does not need to be stated how important a quality fire is. A proper fire isn't just a useful tool in cold climates for warmth, it is also invaluable in warm climates for cooking game, cleansing water, making tools and locating help for rescue. Making a fire without flint, matches or a lighter is a skill that can only come from experience and practice. When entering the wilderness, it is important to always realistically consider your fire making skills. Although the methods in this book will illustrate how to make a fire only from the materials provided in nature, these methods require routine practice. Even with an excess amount of effort, making fire can only happen with the proper technique and materials.

Before making fire, it is important to understand the functionality of the fire triangle. The fire triangle is a hypothetical diagram that illustrates the three necessary components of fire: fuel, oxygen, and heat. All three are necessary to make a fire and a fire cannot exist with anyone missing in the equation. Without fuel and oxygen, the fire cannot be sustained; without heat, the fire cannot ignite.

No matter what method of fire making you are attempting, it starts with tinder. Tinder is the smaller pieces of wood, twigs, barks, grass, and hay that initially light your fire. The drier the tinder the more likely it will catch a spark and light into a full fire. The success of your fire is dependent on finding the proper tinder that is fibrous enough to oxygenate properly as it burns. Your tinder needs to be small enough to ignite a single spark. If your tinder is too big or wet, it will not light and you will not have a fire. Most tree barks, particularly ones with white hues, have natural oils in them that ignite and burn well making them excellent tinder when shredded by hands into small thin pieces. Dry leaves, if available, also make extremely good tinder. However, finding leaves dry enough can be a challenge in some climates or areas that do not receive enough sunlight to dry them properly.

To ignite your tinder, you will need a piece of metal or flint. Since these can be hard to locate in nature, you should always carry a pocket knife that has a sturdy file or flint attached to it. Generating your first spark will always be the biggest challenge in any fire making setting and takes practice. If you are in a wilderness setting and don't have a flint stone, you need to locate a stone that has silica in it. Silica is the combustible material in flint that has a white hue. If you are able to find one after hitting it repeatedly with another stone, you should be able to generate a spark. To light your tinder with a flint stone or steel, you will have to dig an indentation in the earth to protect it from the wind, and then strike your stone slightly above it in order for the tinder to light. If you dig your indentation too far into the earth, the spark will be starved of oxygen and you will not be able to maintain a fire once you do get the tinder to light. If you can successfully light the tinder, slowly place bigger and bigger pieces of tinder on it until the fire can sustain bigger pieces of fuel.

If you do not have a flint or steal and cannot find one, you should attempt to construct a bow drill to ignite a spark. Bow drills are a powerful fire-starting tool that is completely dependent on the proper construction and materials. This construction is made out of a fireboard, a drill, a handhold and a bow. To make the bow, remove a shoelace and tie one end of a pliable stick to the other end so that it has enough tension to make a bow with a defiant capital D shape. Your fireboard with being constructed out of a flat piece of wood that is dry enough to generate heat once we start applying friction to it. Your drill will also be a strong dry branch, that has a tapered tip that can dig into your fireboard to make a notch. The straighter this branch is the more functional the final product will be. And finally, you will need a hand hold that can be anything to place between your hand and the drill while you place pressure on the spinning drill.

This construction works by wrapping your drill tightly in the string of the bow and placing the tip of the drill against the fireboard. When you move the bow back and forth while applying pressure over the spinning drill with your hand hold, the friction on the fire board will now make an ember. Once the construction makes an ember, you can transfer it over to your tinder to ignite a fire. A thick green leave or another piece of wood can be ideal for transporting the ember. Do not use a stone because the cold temperature of a rock can diffuse the ember. If your fireboard is only smoking and not generating an ember, try making an indentation on your fireboard that provided the opportunity for an ember to fall through the notch your drill has made. This fire-starting method

takes time and the proper resources but has been proven
to work.

CHAPTER 3

FINDING WATER AND FOOD IN THE WILD

Tips for finding food

Keep it simple: First things first, if you can start a fire and catch something with either feathers or fur, you don't need to think twice about eating it. This does not include scavenger animals, however, as anything that eats dead flesh could be host to a variety of diseases you can be sure you want no part of. To make sure that you cook the meet properly, you are going to want to cut into the raw meat before you start cooking it, so you know what color it was before you started. You will know the meat is safe to eat when none of the inside of the meat retains its original color.

Cooking an animal will make it safe to eat, but only if the animal was in a generally healthy state, to begin with. As such, you are going to want to take tie prior to killing the animal to observe it in its unagitated state and ensure that it acts the way you would expect such an animal to. If you notice the animal experiencing any type of odd behavior, then this is could be a sign of a potentially serious illness which means you should avoid it no matter what. While you can technically eat about 70 percent of any animal you kill, if you don't make a habit of such things you are going to definitely find it easier to stick to the primary cuts of meet you are familiar with. Finally, even after you cook the meat you should only store it for about 48 hours unless you are someplace extremely cold.

Seafood: Being lost near a body of waters means that you should never have to worry about a reliable source of protein, as longa s you approach the situation correctly. First and foremost, however, it is extremely dangerous to eat fish that live in polluted water which means that you need to be extremely sure of your surroundings before you start fishing. While it is obviously possible to eat raw fish, you never know what type of parasites or bacteria might be living in the fish to start, which means that you are going to want to eat all your fish cooked, no mater what.

In fact, it is actually illegal to serve fresh fish raw until after it has been frozen to ensure all the various bacteria and parasites are removed. If you find yourself fishing in a saltwater body of water, then you are going to want to ensure you get out into the ocean proper to do your fishing. This is crucial as many types of fish that live either near the shore or in a reef are known to carry ciguatera, which can be dangerous when consumed by humans. This goes for fish of any size, as long as it lives on the reef or near the shore.

When fishing further out to see, you are going to want to avoid cowfish, oilfish, red snapper, jack, porcupine fish, trigger fish, puffer fish, and thorn fish because these fish have poisonous flesh. Crustaceans such as shrimp and crayfish are safe to eat as long as they are cooked thoroughly. Mollusks such as octopus and shellfish are also safe. Just note that mussels in tropical areas during summer could be dangerous to consume, as well as any shellfish that stays above water during a high tide.

Looking outside the normal spectrum: If more traditional supplies of meat are unavailable in the area you find yourself in, this does not mean you can lay off of the protein, especially in a strenuous situation. This means you may need to resort to eating insects and other small animals you might not consider traditional food sources. Many insects can be dangerous, so you should avoid eating spiders, caterpillars, brightly colored insects, flies, mosquitos, ticks, and adult insects that sting and bite. Worms are safe to eat, just place them in a container of clean water and they will wash themselves out. Remember, insects that have hard shells on the outside must be cooked first before consuming, others can be consumed raw.

Amphibians: Salamanders and frogs are both safe to eat, though it is important that you are very clear on the difference between toads and frogs as frogs are good eating and toads are poisonous. The easiest way to tell the difference between a toad and a frog is that a toad is almost always more brightly colored and those that are poisonous tend to have an X-shaped pattern on its back. Frogs also have long, thing legs while toads tend to be stout and short. Finally, a frog will hop, and a toad will crawl. Frogs a typically be found in the shallows near bodies of water.

Plants: If you come across a plant that you want to eat, but you are unsure if it is actually edible, the first thing you will need to do is to rub it on your skin. If nothing happens after five minutes, crush a small amount of it between your fingers so it produces a liquid and then rub that liquid on your skin. If this also yields no negative results then the next thing you will want to do is press it to your lips, wait, put it in your mouth, wait and then finally chew up the plant but make sure not to swallow it. If you still do not feel that anything is wrong, then you can swallow only a tiny amount of the plant and then let it digest completely for about 12 hours. After that try eating a larger amount and waiting again before tentatively considering the experiment a success.

When it comes to using this method, it is important to keep in mind that if during any part of the experiment, you feel a burning sensation, or feel ill after swallowing anything then you are going to want to immediately discontinue all testing and induce vomiting if you swallowed more than you should have. Before starting this test, you will also want to go a full eight hours without eating anything first to ensure you get the most accurate results possible. Cook the plants first, if possible, as some plants will lose their toxicity when cooked.

Berries: Many berries are poisonous while many more are good to eat. Unfortunately, unless you are a berry expert, you should make it a habit of sticking to raspberries and blackberries as they are the most distinct of the bunch. If you are in a life or death situation you can perform the plant test on a single berry to start, before increasing from there if you don't notice any ill effects for at least 12 hours.

Fungi: Just like berries, mushrooms can either be deadly or extremely benign. While this isn't true for all mushrooms, generally speaking, you can look at the bottom of the cap and if it is white or producing any type of liquid then you want to leave it alone. Red mushrooms should also be avoided at all costs. If you are left with no choice but to eat a mushroom, start with the plant test, even if it seems benign, and wait 12 hours before increasing dosages. Always cook all mushrooms before eating them for the best results as well.

Water

Above all else, what you need to survive in the wilderness is water. It doesn't matter where you are or where you are going if there is a chance you might end up staying for longer than intended, do yourself a favor and bring plenty of water along for the ride. Nevertheless, even if you take precautions, you will likely find yourself in need of more water if you end up in a true emergency situation which is where the following tips are sure to come in handy.

Water flows downhill: Water will naturally follow the path of least resistance which means that if you are looking for water you are going to want to start from the lowest point around. If you find the bed of a pond that has sense dried up, you can often find water waiting below the surface if you just dig down a little bit. If you can make it to a layer of mud, then you will know that you are close to water.

Always clean it: The only time you should ever risk drinking water before you have purified it is if it is flowing freely, never risk drinking from the shallows as doing so will only lead you to contracting illnesses that are going to make it even harder for you to remain hydrated. The easiest way to purify water is to create a basic filter which can be done by starting with a wet cloth. You then cover it with a layer of charcoal, cleaned gravel, and fresh grass. This allows for four separate layers of filtering and will work on water that you know not to be actively contaminated with anything you don't want to consume.

The grass will remove all the major pollutants, while the gravel, charcoal and wet cloth remove smaller microns of irritants that could make you sick. To activate it, simply hold the filter over a container that you are going to store water in and then poor it through. When possible, you are going to want to start with this method before then boiling the water for 60 seconds. Don't worry for boiling for longer than this as if it wasn't enough to take down the bacteria living in the water then extra heat won't affect it.

Once you have boiled the water, the next thing you will want to do is to purify it chemically if possible. If you have them, a very small amount of bleach or iodine are great for this and all you will need to add is about four drops of these chemicals per quart of cold or murky water, and if you have warm or clear water then you will just need two drops. Give the water a shake and let it sit for about half an hour. If you want to be extra safe you could put that water into a clear plastic water bottle and let it sit in the sun for a few hours as this will cause it to vaporize and then condense again leaving the remaining water as pure as possible.

If you are heading off somewhere where you might need to clean your own water, then investing in a steripen might be a wise choice. A steripen purifies water by emitting an ultraviolet like that kills 99.9 percent of all bacteria rendering virtually any type of water drinkable in seconds. While it may be difficult to work through all of these steps when you haven't any water in 48 hours and you see it there sitting in front of you, it is important to ignore the urge until it is safe to do so. Giving in at this stage will almost certainly lead to diarrhea which will dehydrate you even faster and leave you in a life-threatening situation.

Know your enemy: The three primary waterborne illnesses to look out for include giardia, cryptosporidium, and E. coli. Giardia and cryptosporidium are both parasites unlike E. coli, which is a type of bacteria. Symptoms of these conditions are abdominal cramps, watery stools, bloating, lack of appetite, fever, and vomiting. These conditions are also hard to detect early on because you do not start to get symptoms until a few days after ingesting contaminated water.

Broaden your search: While existing bodies of water are the most obvious choice, if you find yourself without access to one of them, then there are still other options that are available to you. Tree tapping is always an option, though any water that comes from trees is going to contain high amounts of sugar which can harm your body if consumed exclusively. To pull water from a tree, all you need to do is take a knife and dig out a small hole. You should aim to keep the hole as small as possible because it will permanently damage the tree.

You will know you have dug the whole deep enough when it starts leaking water. Once this occurs you will want to take a small piece of wood and shape it, so it is about the same dimensions as a pencil but sharpened on both ends. You will then want to find a rock and use it to hammer the piece of wood into the hole at an angle, so the water can freely drip from it.

With this done, all you need to do is attach your canteen or another water container to the bottom of the stick and wait. It is important to keep in mind that it will take most of the day to fill up a canteen using this method and, even then, it only works with birch, sycamore, maple and other similar trees.

Ferns of all types are also a good source of water. To access it, all you need to do is dig around its roots until you find something that looks similar to a potato, that is about the size of a gumball. Crack this open and you should find enough water to sate your thirst for a short time.

Another good choice is what is known as a solar still as it will allow you to collect a fair amount of water overnight. All you need to get this up and running is a container to store the water in, some fresh leaves and a plastic bag. To get started, all you need to do is dig a hole in the ground that is about as deep as the length of your arm. The hole should also be wide enough to fit a pair of basketballs. From there, you will need to find some fresh leaves and crush them gently before setting them in the bottom of the hole. It is important that these leaves are as clean as possible and from a plant that you know not to be poisonous as you will be drinking from them directly.

With this done, you will then need to place the container on top of the leaves. Keep the container small, it should only cover about half of the total available space. With this done, you will then need to cover the hole with something plastic, before pinning it in place with a number of heavy rocks. Once the plastic is secure, you will then place another rock in the center that is heavy enough to weight the plastic down in the area of the container. With this done, the moisture that collects on the leaves overnight will be heated by the morning sun, causing it to rise as condensation. This liquid will get caught in the plastic and then drip into the container where it will be completely cleaned and ready to drink.

Another way to accomplish the same thing is to find a tree branch or bush that is full of leaves and then cover it with plastic to get the same results. Again, always make sure the solar still is directly in contact with the sun and the plant you choose has already proven to be nontoxic.

Finally, if you have an extra piece of clothing handy, you can tie it around your ankles and walk through a field or patch of tall grass early in the morning and collect the moisture from them. While this won't be enough to keep you hydrated in the long-term, it should be enough to keep you going while you work on a more permanent

solution.

CHAPTER 4

FINDING HELP

Before heading out into the wilderness, regardless of how long you expect to be gone or where you are going, it is always important to let at least two people know where you are going and when you plan on getting back. It doesn't matter how competent you feel about yourself or your activities, this small bit of preparation could easily save your life. Along similar lines, if you are planning an extended stay in the great outdoors, plan on checking in with someone in the outside world at least once a week.

If you do find yourself in an emergency situation, assuming you are not in any immediate danger, the first thing you will want to do is think about how you are going to get in touch with the outside world. If you are relatively close to civilization, then your phone might still be in working order, if you are traveling off the beaten path then a long rang walkie-talkie or radio might be a better choice. Before heading out into the wilderness for multiple days, take the time to determine what level of communication is available in the area, you will be glad you did.

In order to take advantage of potential rescuers, it is important to be able to give them as much information as possible when you do get in touch with them, which means doing your research beforehand and never straying from your planned excursion unless it is unavoidable. When you get out of your car and again when you reach your destination or make camp for the night you should mark that spot onto a map. Then, using a compass, jot down your general direction and any other coordinates you can muster. Also, note any major landmarks that you pass by, especially anything you feel will be noticeable from the air.

What to do when lost

If you find yourself lost in the wilderness, then you are going to want to keep in mind the acronym STOP as doing so will make your situation far more manageable.

Stay put: While it can be hard to sit around and wait for help to find you, if you are lost in an unfamiliar area this is just what you should do. Staying in one place will make it easier for others to find you, especially if you have no real idea of how to reach civilization which means you could just as easily be hurting your situation as helping it. Keep in mind, if you do decide to press your luck, each step you take outside of the area you told others you would be in takes you another step away from anywhere your preparations might be useful. The only time when this might not be the case is if you are close to something that will allow you to dramatically improve your vantage point which can make it easier for you to take stock of your situation and also make you more visible to rescue attempts from the air.

T: Think about everything you remember about where you have come from. You never know what details might help a rescue team find you or even help you reorient yourself so that you realize you weren't actually lost as well which is why it is important to take stock of everything you remember from the point you knew where you were to the point you found yourself lost as quickly as possible. Short term memories fade quickly, and small details, especially those you weren't paying attention to in the first place, fade more quickly still; these are the details that can literally save your life so do everything you can to solidify them in your mind ASAP.

O: Observe your surroundings. Once you have taken stock of how you ended up in your current situation the next thing that you will want to do is consider the area you currently find yourself in, specifically anything that appears as though it was made or altered by humans or any new landmarks. If you find something that is manmade then the odds of someone coming along will increase exponentially and you will have even more of a reason not to leave the area and additional landmarks will make it easier for a rescue team to find you if you do, make contact with someone.

P: Plan out what you will do next. If you do find yourself in an emergency situation it is important to take the time to consider all of your various potential courses of action. The seriousness of your current situation will radically change the next steps you have to take and planning before going off half-cocked.

After you have made it through all of the acronym, you should then have a pretty good idea of where you are in relation to where you started out from. However, if you feel as though you are extremely lost, then the best choice is always going to be staying put and creating signals to help others find you (as discussed later in this chapter). If you are certain you now know where you got off track, you can instead try and find your way back to safety.

Above all else, you need to ensure that your first course of action is not to become any more lost than you already are. This means you should start by creating a reference point, either a natural formation or something you create, to ensure you won't forget where you came from. With that done, you will then want to leave a clear trail so that you can find your way back to where you started from, at the very least. You can make a trail by break twigs and branches along your route, by leaving things from your pack along as you go, or even by dragging a stick along behind you as you walk. With this done, if you realize you took another wrong turn, it will then be extremely easy to backtrack and try again.

Signal for help

If you have decided that your best course of action is to stay put, then you will want to focus on covering all the core survival basics as you never know how long you might have to remain in the area. Assuming you are not in any immediate danger, however, the first thing you are going to want to do is create some sort of signal that will show any who happens by that things are not as they should be.

Visual cues: Assuming you can create one, there is nothing better than a signal fire to indicate that a human is somewhere they shouldn't be. The best type of signal fire is going to produce, thick black smoke, the darker the better, to ensure that it can be easily spotted from a distance. To make this smoky dream a reality, you are going to want to start with a large normal fire. Take care not to build something you can't control, however, as starting a forest fire is the last thing you want to do. You will want to create this fire in the most visible spot possible, so the smoke is visible from the maximum possible distance.

After you have the fire burning strong, you are going to want to add in anything you can find that it will help it to burn nice and black. The darkest smoke of all is going to come from motor oil, plastic or brake fluid. If you have any of these available, ration them until you believe that you see signs of life on the horizon to maximize your odds of being seen. Ideally, however, you will be able to find a steady supply of fresh, green tree branches, the fresher the better. If you even have to venture away from your signal fire, take care to leave a note or some indication that you have not yet been rescued to ensure that anyone who stops doesn't get the wrong idea.

While not as useful as a full signal fire, you should always carry a mirror with you if you are planning to venture into the wilderness as it is a compact way to ensure you can always get someone's attention, even at a distance. If you find yourself without a mirror, you can also use tinfoil an aluminum can, or anything else shiny to attract attention. At night, a laser pointer or flashlight can also be a literal lifesaver.

Audio cues: Yelling and screaming becomes practically useless if your rescuer is more than a few hundred yards away. As such, it is always a good idea to stow an emergency whistle in with your camping gear to not only save the strain on your voice, but also travel a much greater distance as well. If possible, gunfire will also tell someone else that you are in the area beyond a shadow of a doubt. When it comes to signaling for help in this fashion, you are going to want to repeat your signal in groups of three short blasts, that are each about five seconds apart. This will not only tell others that you need help but will give them time to set up an audio cue to let you know they heard you.

CHAPTER 5

SURVIVAL FIRST AID

If you find yourself in need of first aid during an emergency situation, the first thing you should keep in mind is that you need to stay calm. Regardless of what trauma you are suddenly facing, losing your cool is only going to serve to exacerbate the issue, guaranteed. On the other hand, by remaining calm, you are helping to ensure that you don't end up accidentally doing something foolish that will make the situation worse. In this type of situation, it is important to keep in mind that you are the only person who can ensure you make it through this situation in one piece which means you need to stop worrying about what's happened and start worrying about how you can fix it.

Broken bones and cuts: Scratches, bites and minor cuts should always be cleaned out with clean water as well as a disinfectant, if possible, before stopping the bleeding as best you can. Make sure to change the bandage every four hours, or more frequently if you have reason to believe the injury might be infected. If you are dealing with a broken or fractured bone, the situation can easily be more serious. You will want to first stop any bleeding using a tourniquet before following that up with a splint.

If you are dealing with a deeper cut that doesn't want to stop bleeding, you will want to use something that has been sterilized to apply pressure directly to the wound. If this is not available, then you will want to use homemade dressing instead as anything that is not sterilized could end up infecting the wound. Still, if you are out of options, a dirty shirt is still a good deal better than not bleeding to death. If you can't apply enough pressure to get the bleeding to stop you will want to use a tourniquet instead.

Creating a tourniquet: While the use of a tourniquet has critics on both sides of the issue, the truth of the matter is that as long as the tourniquet is applied properly and not left on unnecessarily then it can easily save a person's life with little to no negative side effects. While concerns of nerve damage and limb loss are not unfounded, recent studies show that less than half of one percent of all people who are treated for blood loss via the use of a tourniquet require limb amputation because of the tourniquet and less than two percent of all people experience any type of nerve damage. Damage from prolonged tourniquet use doesn't begin for upwards of two hours, and upwards of eight hours of continuous use are required before amputation becomes a realistic option.

While a professional tourniquet is nice if you can get one, it is hardly something you are going to want to keep in your pack on regular basis, especially when there are so many other useful things you could use instead. Easy tourniquet alternatives include a belt, the sleeve of a long-sleeved shirt, the laces from your shoes, the strap of a bra, basically anything you can pull tight and trust not to loosen on its own.

With the tourniquet in hand, you are also going to need something to keep it tight, which is known as a torsion device. This can be anything that is long and thin, but still strong enough to not break under pressure. Remember, you can use a tourniquet on any of your limbs, but never on your neck, this should be self-explanatory, but people are rarely thinking clearly in a crisis.

To us the tourniquet successfully, you will want to wrap it around the afflicted limb about two inches closer to your core than where the injury is. When lining up the tourniquet, ensure that you avoid any major arteries or joints. If you aren't sure about your placement, move closer to your core as opposed to further away. Once it has been positioned properly, you will then want to tie it in place using a single overhand knot. Finally, you will want to set the torsion device on top of the knot and then tie it in place using either an overhand knot or a square knot.

Creating a splint: If you find yourself in need of a splint, the first thing you will need to do is locate something that is rigid enough to keep the fractured bone stabilized. Wood is the most commonly used component, though rolled up newspaper will work in a pinch. When you need to secure the split, you can use any of the items you would use for a tourniquet as it can serve the same purpose.

Before creating a splint, it is important to stop any bleeding as this is always going to be the top priority. It is also important to try and avoid moving the person in need of a split, or at least the damaged area, as much as possible as doing so can easily cause the injury to become more severe. While keeping these things in mind, you are also going to want to set the splint in such a way that it can reach above the afflicted area and align with the joints on either side.

For example, if you needed to make a splint for your forearm, you would want the split to reach all the way from your wrist to your elbow. When you tie on the split you are going to want to ensure that it is tight enough to prevent unwanted movement while at the same time not being tight enough to prevent blood flow.

If you need to put a splint on your hand or someone else's, the first thing you will want to do is place something soft in the palm and have them ball the hand into a loose fist. After the fingers have closed around the object, the next thing you will want to do is wrap the entire hand in a large cloth, only leaving the fingertips exposed. This cloth should move in a horizontal fashion across the hand, starting at the thumb and moving directly towards the pinky. Once this is done, you will then want to bind the hand using extra ties, taking care to bind it loosely enough that you don't cut off circulation.

Burns: To treat a burn, you have to identify the cause of the burn and act accordingly. Burns from the cold temperature should be warmed by placing the area of the burn in warm water or by blowing warm air on the burn. Burns from hot liquid should be cooled by running cold water over it for 10-20 minutes and never use ice. If someone is burned from being electrocuted, then you should separate them from the current and immediately check for a pulse and apply CPR if necessary. With the torsion device in place, you will then want to rotate it, so the tourniquet tightens against the limb just until the point that the bleeding stops, it is important to not put more constraints on the limb than necessary so stop the moment the blood loss subsides. Finally, you will want to ensure the torsion device is going to remain in place by taking the ends of the second knot and tying it to the limb and the tourniquet respectively.

Chocking: Choking can be a particularly dangerous accident if you are stranded in the wilderness. First aid for choking begins with five back thrusts, which can be done using the palm of your hand to strike between the choking victim's shoulder blades. Once this is done, you will want to perform a series of five abdominal thrusts, also known as the Heimlich maneuver. To perform this maneuver correctly, you need to stand behind the choking victim before wrapping them in your arms, so your hands line up with their belly button. Once you are in the position you will want to pull upward at an angle in short bursts and repeat as needed.

CPR: Cardiopulmonary Resuscitation should be performed immediately if someone has little nor no pulse and is unresponsive. This could be a result of drowning, electrocution, poisoning, or fainting. The first step is to call for medical help immediately, if possible and then begin CPR. By performing CPR, you are allowing oxygenated blood to flow around the body of the victim. Without this oxygenated blood the brain is not receiving any oxygen and in only a matter of minutes, the victim's brain will start to receive serious damage. It only takes eight minutes without blood flow for the brain to die.

The first thing you are going to want to do is to position the person in need of CPR on their back with their head facing the sky and tilt their head at an angle to ensure that their airway is unrestricted. You will then want to put your hands on their sternum and, with your arms straight, push onto the person's sternum 30 times in a quick manner. This step is called the chest compressions and the amount of strength used should vary depending on who is receiving CPR chest compressions should be administered at a rate of 100 pumps per minute. For young children and old people, you should use little force as their ribs may break. When performing chest compressions your patient's ribs may break during the process so as soon as you start hearing the cracking you want to immediately stop the compressions for a few seconds and then resume with the chest compressions.

After performing 30 chest compressions the next step is to breathe for the person. First, you want to make sure that their chin is up, and head tilted back to clear all airways into the victim's lungs. Next, pinch the nostrils and make an airtight seal with your lips onto your patient's and breathe into them. You should also keep an eye on the chest of the victim and see if it is rising up and down as you breathe into them. You need to apply two breaths and immediately start doing chest compressions again. This should be repeated over and over until help arrives or the victim starts to respond and is breathing on their own.

Venom or poison: If you discover that you or someone you are traveling with has ingested a poison substance, then it is important to take action immediately, as time is of the essence. First things first, you will need to recognize the symptoms as someone who is fighting off poison will often behave erratically, act confused, or have trouble breathing. If left untreated, they may begin vomiting and develop redness or other discoloration around their hands and face.

If traditional medical treatment is not an option, the first thing you are going to want to do is to ensure you induce vomiting in the afflicted party. This can be difficult if the afflicted individual is already feeling the effects of the poison but is crucial if you want to prevent things from getting worse. You will then want to rise the mouth of the victim out with water. If the poison entered through the skin, then you will need to rinse the affected area continuously for at least 15 minutes. If the poison comes into contact with the eyes directly, wash them out with continuously flowing water for 30 minutes or more.

If the poison comes from a spider or insect, then the first thing you will want to do is get away from the nesting area before removing any stingers that may have stuck in the skin. You will then need to clean out the area using soap and water, before applying an ice pack or cold water to reduce the swelling. If the point of contact was on a limb, keep that limb close to the ground to reduce the rate at which the venom spreads.

When it comes to dealing with snakes, it is important to keep in mind that some are completely harmless, while others can kill you with little more than a look. The primary stakes to look out for in the continental US are the cottonmouth, rattlesnake and copperhead. If you find yourself fending off a snakebite, you will know if it injected venom into you if you feel signs of fainting, dizziness, weakness, nausea, swelling, vomiting, convulsions, loss of muscle control, rapid pulse or diarrhea.

If possible, you are going to want to kill the snake and bring it with you or take a picture of it so that you can show it to a medical professional assuming you are able to get to one in time. This is critical as every snake has a different type of venom, which means the antivenom required is different as well. If you don't have any other options, you are going to want to quickly make a small cut in the skin above the location of the bite so that you can attempt to suck the venom out. Be careful if you do so, however, as if you swallow you will be worse off than you were to start.

In the US, all the snakes you need to worry about, with the exception of the coral snake are what are known as pit vipers. This means you just need to be on the lookout for a thick snake with a large head and pupils that are shaped like slits. They also have two indentions on their nose, known as heat pits, which is a good indication that it is poisonous. Generally speaking, if you come across a thin snake then it is unlikely to be poisonous. The coral snake is an exception to just about every rule regarding poisonous snakes, which means that you want to remember that if the pattern is red and black, it's safe Jack; meanwhile, if its red and yellow then it could kill you, fellow.

CONCLUSION

Thank you for making it through to the end of *Survival Skills: Basic Survival Skills Everyone Should Know*, let's hope it was informative and able to provide you with all of the tools you need to achieve your goals, whatever it is that they may be. Just because you've finished this book doesn't mean there is nothing left to learn on the topic, expanding your horizons is the only way to find the mastery you seek.

Just because you have finished this book and have a general idea of how to handle yourself in a wilderness survival scenario doesn't mean that you can be lax when it comes to planning your various nature excursions. Proper preparedness is going to be the key to coming through an unexpected emergency scenario unscathed 100 percent of the time. If you don't take the time to plan ahead successfully when venturing off the beaten path you could very well literally be taking your life into your hands.

If you do find yourself in a survival situation, the best thing you can do is stay calm and take stock of your immediate situation. If you can determine a list of primary needs that should be addressed, then you are already well on your way to improve your odds of survival significantly. Many situations can be deceptively dangerous and keeping your guard up at all time is going to be crucial to your success, you never know when being hyper-alert might be the difference between life and death. As a member of the dominant species on the planet, you are capable of living in even the world's most deadly conditions, never forget this and you can survive anything.

Finally, if you found this book useful in any way, a review on Amazon is always appreciated!